# *Communicating with your Elderly Loved Ones:*

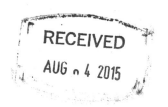
## *Practical Recommendations for Interacting at Home or at Eldercare Centers*

### *Joanne Hughes, M.A.*
### *Rita Miller, R.N.*

1stBooks – rev. 7/9/01

# Table of Contents:

# About the Authors:

**Joanne Hughes, M.A.**, is the president of BCW Inc., Business Communication Workshops, a firm specializing in communication programs, seminars and speeches. In addition, Hughes is currently Adjunct Professor of Communication subjects at Mount Saint Mary College, Newburgh, NY. Her earlier books include *Effective Communication* for NYNEX and *Effective Presentation* for GE. She has written over 40 programs in business management and communication with several on video and audiotape as well as many articles and papers.

**Rita Miller, R.N.**, began her nursing career at Mary Immaculate Hospital in Jamaica, New York. After serving in Geriatric Home Care, she met the needs of elderly patients in a highly praised retirement home in Middletown, NY, becoming Director of Nursing and Assistant Administrator. Retiring from active nursing in 1994, she is volunteering at Hospice of Orange County.

# FOREWORD

Elizabeth was lying in her invalid's bed, pale and unmoving. Her eyes were open and staring but she didn't respond to her only daughter bending over her. The younger woman had been told to use smiles and nods and gentle language by her friend, a nurse in a home for the elderly; so the younger woman chatted animatedly with the virtually comatose little lady for several minutes but without result.

Then suddenly, the 83-year-old woman turned her face directly toward her daughter's and said with great warmth: "I love you."

Elizabeth was my mother and those were the last words she spoke to me. You can imagine how I treasure that moment. Frankly, I'm not sure I could have created the climate which released my poor, senile mother for that brief second of contact if it had not been for my friend, Rita Miller.

It was Rita who had been advising me for the several years while Elizabeth had been sliding into senility and loss of vital functions.

Over dinners, during social occasions, on the phone, I would relate some new and surprising twist in my mother's decline for which I was totally unprepared, and Rita would smile her sharing smile and offer some good practical advice for me to follow in this next phase.

It was this experience that has triggered our collaboration on this little book. This is a conversation between two old friends on a subject very close to our hearts.

# 1. *WHAT THE BOOK IS ABOUT*

## * *Conversations between Two Friends*

Joanne: "I recall a statement of yours when you were Director of Nursing at that Middletown Retirement Home. You said it was at the heart and soul of caring for the elderly and I have never forgotten it. You said it so simply:
'We must treat them as we would treat our own mothers.'"

Rita: "You remembered that! I'm flattered. Well, we had always felt that we had been invited into *their* home, even if it was a facility for the aged, and in truth, we were *their* guests, coming to their homes to help them."

Joanne: "I didn't forget because it was so moving to hear you as a professional caregiver speak like that. Some healthcare pros guard their feelings so strongly and protectively that they seem to be losing the humane touch. Yet you offered the same degree of compassion to your patients as you were offering me, a friend of many years, in your advice about my parents."

Rita: "Often healthcare professionals don't want to work in nursing homes because their reason for coming into the medical field is to cure or make the sick or injured well. In geriatric service, you've got to change your attitude from 'make everybody well' to 'accept the inevitable and make each person as comfortable as possible. For me, doing that particular service with the elderly gives me so much satisfaction and sometimes even joy."

Joanne: "That's so like you, Rita. In my case, I was only trying to keep from doing the wrong thing to my mother and maybe find the right thing. So to hear you say: 'We want to treat them as we would our own mothers;' — that held special meaning for me."

Rita: "I'm glad I could help. There are practices which really help."

Joanne: "I want to share those ideas in this book."

## *Love our Elderly and be Good to Ourselves

Joanne: "Essentially, what we want this book to do is this:

— Encourage greater compassion toward our elderly by caregivers;

— Develop techniques and devices to ease the burden of caregiving.

Rita: "We're addressing home care of the elderly primarily?"

Joanne: 'Yes, although your recommendations can be used across the board."

Rita: 'Well, anything I found useful was learned both in and out of the nursing home environment; so the lessons have merit in both areas.

Joanne: "All I know is that you helped me so much with my parents in their home care. I don't know what I would have done without you."

Rita: "These close family ties are at once a blessing and a tremendous difficulty, Joanne. As you know, I have worked with the population of a retirement home for years. Yet, in many ways, the care that was really very hard for me was the care I gave to my own father, as he was dying, and then again to my terminally ill mother-in-law in her confused state.

"In fact, I really found it much harder to care for my loved ones in a home setting than it had been previously in a professional setting. It was far more emotionally draining. I suspect that it was the same for you with your mother and now with your elderly father."

Joanne: "I've got to tell you that I find it so helpful to hear you say that. Maybe there's hope for me yet."

Rita: "We're all human in our reactions to old age, especially up close. Those with good hearts just try to do the best they can."

## 2. *PLAN IN ADVANCE*

### *Encourage Elderly to Share Their Ideas*

Joanne: "For the purposes of this book, Rita, I'd like to concentrate on eldercare in the home, although I'm aware that you could talk with me for days on all phases of adult health care."

Rita: "Well, I've been in this field a long time. I've just been paying attention!"

Joanne: "Yes, you have! Now let me ask you what your first recommendation would be for a compassionate caregiver?"

Rita: "I believe we must become aware of the need to share ideas with those to whom we would give care — early on. By talking openly with us, they can have valuable input into their own care while they're still mentally and physically able to let us know what their feelings and decisions might be."

Joanne: "That makes sense, although I think many people are afraid to approach communication with their elderly relatives or friends because they don't want to face the reality of advancing old age. Or they're not sure how receptive they will be to the topic. After all, I know people who won't make a will!"

Rita: "Yes, it's true; yet it's so important to start these exchanges about what might lie in the future when our relatives or elderly friends, and even ourselves, are younger."

## *Question Sensitively

Joanne: "Okay then, just what questions would you ask in these touchy exchanges? What information are you trying to establish?"

Rita: "Try questions like: 'What do they expect us to do? What are their expectations of us as their children? Could they conceive of living with us? Would they think about entering a retirement home? What are their expectations of care if they were to become seriously ill or incapacitated?"

Joanne: "In other words, establish a dialogue?

Rita: "Exactly."

Joanne:    "When I teach my courses in Interpersonal Communication,  the experts always recommend the introduction of shared experiences as a way to encourage another to open up.  In this case, I expect that questions about their earlier experiences with their own parents or elderly relatives would be a good jumping-off place for this dialogue."

Rita: "No question.  Mature people love to talk about the culture and the values which produced them,  so channeling the questioning in that direction should prove fruitful."

Joanne:  "Let's put our heads together to come up with a list of appropriate questions to elicit the reactions needed to come to understand just what it is our loved ones want and need from us for their future planning."

Rita:  "Good idea."

# *Checklist for Understanding

The entire point of this checklist is to encourage dialogue between people looking at the later years of their lives and the people who will love and care for  them during those years.  Misunderstandings can happen unless expectations are shared.  Use these questions or create your own.  Make it abundantly clear that this is a first conversation only, and other talks will  follow in the coming months.  Try to speak from their vantage point. Tell them this is a form of brainstorming only.

Let's talk about your grandparents.  How long did they live?

Were they able to stay in their own homes in their later years or did they have to find alternatives?  What were the alternatives in those days?   How did your parents handle these situations?   Was there criticism of the way they handled things?

How about your own parents?  Were they long lived?

What were their needs in their later years?  How were they cared for and by whom?   Were there any other members of our family who needed special care?  Aunts, grand-uncles, sisters or brothers?

What were their opinions about nursing homes in those years? Do you think it's the same now? What happened if the elderly relatives suffered a stroke or hip fracture?

Did they believe their children had to care for them in their home environment in old age? Would you change anything about those years?

Were there organizations like Meals on Wheels or Senior Adult Programs or Daytime Nursing Home care in those days? Did any elderly people go to college programs for elderly people then?

Do you know anyone now who was or is in a nursing home or lifecare situation?
What do you think about their experiences?

What kinds of decisions are your long-time friends making now?

What do you think about their choices?

Have you thought about living with family? What are your thoughts on that?
What if your children are unable to physically care for you in your home or in their own home? What are your thoughts on that possible eventuality?

What are your own feelings about nursing homes?

What if there was an emergency happening to you — stroke or heart attack — what then?

Would you like us to join you in looking up information about the many choices out there for older people today: adult residences, lifecare contracts, retirement communities, long-term life insurance?

Have you begun to formulate any plans for the future about issues like that?


How about financial plans?  Has anyone sat down with you to talk about these years of your retirement?


Add your own questions:

## *Be Empathic.*

Joanne: "If families could take this checklist and use it in the early stages of advancing age with their loved ones, it would not only spark dialogue but it would also prevent so much later misunderstanding."

Rita: "Yes, it would also create empathy between both parties while allowing the older people to sense the concerns and affection of the younger group."

Joanne: "Each would need to understand the reactions of the others for maximum communication. Nothing does that better than open conversation without a lot of stress."

Rita: "Unless people think ahead in this way, these conversations happen after someone has fallen or a spouse has died or they've passed the point where they can make decisions. It's so much better to plan ahead."

Joanne: "When you mentioned empathy, I recalled a poignant poem my husband Edward wrote upon seeing the reactions of my elderly father and our young grandson, Steven. It certainly makes one aware of just how tough old age can be and how communication eases the anguish.

## Grandfather and Grandson

You know, Grandpa, said the small boy,
We're really quite a pair.
With Mom and Dad observing us
In troubles that we share.
When dropping food down on the floor
At times throughout a meal,
The looks we get can make us mad;
Ashamed is how we feel.
If we don't get to bathroom,
In time for what needs doing,
We'll hear about our bad mistake;
It really leaves us stewing.
And if we cry or oversleep
Or act with loud emotion,
The adults frown and put us down;
They just don't have a notion!
So we complain and 'miserate,
Each in our special way,
But it makes me feel so good to be
With you along the way.

## * *Ask for Help*

Rita: "Here is the starting point leading to solving eldercare concerns and worries. Brochures and pamphlets of adult residences can be requested by mail from addresses in the phone book. Visits to local eldercare facilities can be planned just to establish the basis for future decisions. Include the older person on these information excursions; truth is better than fear.

"Usually there are local Offices of the Aging; their information can be invaluable as well, helping to identify solutions and alternatives we may not yet know about. Only then can we begin to make a plan of action."

Joanne: "Planning ahead can get very complicated sometimes, especially when it comes to health issues. I remember taking my father for his annual physical. He was beginning to get confused. He was 89 then."

Rita: "He's allowed a little confusion at 89!"

Joanne: "Dressing himself with a time limit had become a problem. When the doctor told him to put on the gown and leave it open in the back, well, that took him a long time and the doctor was waiting to examine him. Things got a little tense. Apparently, no nurse was available either and I didn't think to ask for one."

Rita: "Maybe asking for nursing help is a good rule of thumb in caring for any elderly person."

Joanne: "Believe me I've done that ever since, but not that day. There I was wanting to provide that help, but there was the gender issue with me, the female child of a male relative. I couldn't bring myself to stay in the examining room with him. I just couldn't risk seeing my father naked nor, I suspect, could he have handled my seeing him that way either. So I stood outside the door and called in to him to encourage him as he undressed.

"He managed it all, had his exam, re-dressed himself and came out. Now don't laugh when I tell you that I was exhausted at the end of that."

Rita: "No, I understand; that was hard."

Joanne: "The thing was that when he rejoined me, he said to the doctor:

'She's my nurse.' Well, actually, I didn't like that. I'm not his nurse; I'm his daughter. And while I didn't say anything, it gave me a bad feeling. It goes back to exactly what you've been saying, Rita. He and I had never discussed what my role was going to be with him when he needed care, although there was no question that I would help him were he sick or injured."

Rita: "Yes, but because you and he hadn't talked it over, he'd made a decision unilaterally about his care: 'You are his nurse.' However, that's not what you want to be; that wasn't something you two had an understanding about. And the strength of your reaction shows how much you did need to talk this over with him. The thought of your truly nursing him, without any training or knowledge,...."

Joanne: "...that terrified me."

### *Talk as early as possible*

Rita: "It's an important and sensitive issue. Further, I think that when you talk about these issues of elderly care, Joanne, it shouldn't just begin when they're elderly.

The exchanges should begin in their middle years when all parties can sit down together and talk about the future. When the child becomes an adult, that's when the conversations should begin. That's when the plans for care should be laid down, at least as a starting point."

Joanne: "Starting point. Right. However, circumstances can intervene."

Rita: "That's right. Circumstances change everything. But this way, there's a foundation and an openness between the child and the older relative."

Joanne: "Currently, my father has entered my home at my invitation — but we've never talked it through. I'll try harder to find opportunities to establish more empathy with him. One thing though, we have talked about money."

Rita: "Oh, that's great! There are so many people who can't bring themselves to talk about that. So issues of finance like wills, income, mortgages become forbidden territory even though it is absolutely crucial to all their lives. That's too bad — especially when things start to happen where the parent is spending money unwisely and no provision has been made."

## *Spending Money Unwisely*

Joanne: "Do I know that! My Dad became a victim of unscrupulous mail solicitations and sent $1600 in one year alone to what we regard as false organizations parading as political entities. He was receiving eight to ten pieces of solicitation mail every single day! It confused him terribly, not to mention the expense he incurred."

Rita: "That's just criminal!"

Joanne: "What's worse, we contacted the organizations and the Post Office, and nothing changed! In fact, my husband's name got onto their mailing lists and they solicited him from then on!"

Rita: "What did you do then?"

Joanne: "We went to our attorney with Dad and had him write up a Power of Attorney for us. We then started screening his mail. I don't like it but I really have no choice with these kinds of unethical mail appeals — and his generous heart."

Rita: "So many people have been victimized in this way. Political, social, charitable appeals, and the worst, the Sweepstakes!"

Joanne: "That was the most terrible. One morning, Dad was absolutely convinced that he had won two million dollars. And in his generosity, he was telling people that he would give them some!"

Rita: "That was awful. Of course, it is not that unusual. The way those letters are written makes many older people confused about whether they've won the awards. You know: JANE JONES WINS A MILLION DOLLARS! For people raised to believe in the printed word, it seems like reality. Intervention is so important here."

Joanne: "It just proves that what you're saying is so sound, Rita. We need to try to talk with our parents or relatives early, and if not early, at least, later."

## *Fear of Nursing Homes*

Rita: "During these conversations, some older people will express fears of living in nursing homes. That gives you a chance to go over why they have these fears. For some of them, it's because in their time years before, when they visited their old relatives, they heard or even witnessed some horrible situations."

Joanne: "Things have changed so much since the fifties and sixties."

Rita: "With these conversations, you might be able to take away their fears and help them to find out what today's nursing homes and adult care facilities are really like. Or at the very least, figure out how to work around those fears and reach good decisions."

Joanne: "First step in good communication practice is to have those fears expressed."

Rita: "Yes, and be ready to bolster their courage with reality. Bring along written information like brochures from the Office of the Aging or catalogs, or descriptions of various eldercare housing — anything that gives up-to-date information about today's healthcare for the elderly."

## *Expectations of You as Caregiver

Rita: "It's also important to find out their expectations of you as their caregiver. Do they expect you to take them into your home to the end of their lives? Sometimes there's an expectation like that which the child never knows about. If circumstances dictate and the parent must be put in a nursing home, there's anger and resentment at the child because their parental expectations were not met. Yet often, the child never even knew of these expectations."

Joanne: "Oh, yes, we've run into that through our friends' experiences."

Rita: "Too often."

Joanne: "So you're recommending that people sit down together and explore these expectations?"

Rita: "Yes; they could say: 'I'm reading this book called *Communicating with your Elderly*

*Loved Ones.* It's about caregiving for older people.

It suggests that we talk about some of the issues of caregiving, particularly when people are clear enough to understand each other. It could give us a better idea of what you have in mind for your future. It includes a *Checklist for Understanding* to spark dialogue. Would you like to see it?"

Joanne: "That's a sensible beginning. It is exactly what you and I are trying to do here — as a nurse specializing in Geriatrics and a communication specialist living the experience — to open avenues of communication for the caregiver and the recipient of that care."

Rita: "This is a way to get that dialogue going while creating empathy on both sides right from the beginning."

# 3. *ALLEVIATE ANXIETY*

## *Calming their Fears

Joanne: "You've told me that one of the most important areas you'd like to touch upon in terms of home care for the elderly is that of calming the fears, grounded or groundless, of our family members."

Rita: "Yes, I think recognizing their anxiety and then helping them to control it is extremely important, even to the caregivers who might be very confused by the episodes."

Joanne: "I can remember my mother's periods of anxiety. I didn't always understand them as such. Usually the dementia grabbed my attention and often kept me from looking for the underlying cause."

Rita: "Yes, there is often some emotion under the surface that is prompting the behavior."

Joanne: "The poor woman would pick up on some disturbing thought, and it would grow into something awful. There was one time when she started repeating over and over: 'I think my father is dead, but they're not telling me. I need to know!' And then she'd cry.

"Now the first time you hear something like that it rips your heart out. Of course, by the *tenth* time, you're more irritated than sad. In this instance, we had explained that her father had been dead for over 50 years, yet that didn't seem to help her agitated state. So finally I called you and you told me what to do to help this repetitive questioning."

Rita: "The important thing was to see that the question was immaterial. It was a welling up of fear or anger that was sparking the repetitions. To gentle those feelings with loving attention and a touch of reality would be much more successful than simply informing her of the error of her thoughts."

### * Clarity Cards

Joanne: "Well, your advice worked. What you told me to do was to keep a supply of 3 by 5 inch cards on hand. On the cards, messages could be handwritten to soften the fearful or agitated delusions in my mother's mind. On a card, I wrote a warm, very loving note to her in big letters. It told the truth of her father's long-ago death while re-affirming our affection for her."

Rita: "Do you recall what you said?"

Joanne: "As matter of fact, even after all these years, I do.

*Dearest,*

>*As you know, your wonderful father has been in heaven for 50 years now. He loved you very much just as we do. Don't be feeling bad. He's very happy now.*

>*Love, Your Daughter Joanne*

Rita: "And you say it worked?"

Joanne: "Absolutely. It seemed to answer some need which Mother wasn't expressing or couldn't express. At the same time, for the sake of our sanity, it stopped the incessant repetition, at least, temporarily."

Rita: "Temporarily?"

Joanne: "Well, yes. It rarely worked for good. Usually it would calm her for a period of 20 to 30 minutes, and then she'd ask again after her father.

We would answer in the way you told us: 'Look at your card, Mother. You'll see. Everything's fine.' It was so much easier and less exhausting to say that sentence than to reiterate the emotional message again and again."

Rita: "How long did she have the ability to read the cards?"

Joanne: "Almost to the end. It was amazing that even though her logical or memory capacities were short circuited, her ability to read remained for such a long time compared to other skills."

Rita: "Complete with short-term comprehension?"

Joanne: "Amazingly — Yes. Tell me, in your experience, was her ability unusual or an isolated case?"

Rita: "Not at all unusual. It surprises us in nursing care to observe how long the learned reading response remains with the elderly person. It's very compassionate to use this gift to bring some peace into the mind of the older person."

## * *Use of stickies*

Joanne: "There was another suggestion you gave me that also helped to curtail anxiety: the use of those tiny stamp-size notes with the sticky tape on the back."

Rita: "Oh, yes, they are so helpful. What we would do with them was to place them on the mirror the night before an event that the older person was going to attend. You are aware of how any change in schedule can agitate and stress."

Joanne: "My father sometimes becomes cranky when he's going to have lunch with old friends. You'd think he'd be pleased, but I suspect he's afraid he'll forget something — or forget the event itself."

Rita: "Oh, yes. Again fear is the culprit. Anything we can do to control the fear by thinking ahead helps them and us."

Joanne: "What would you do?"

Rita: "The other nurses and I would help them make decisions about what would be worn on the day ahead, and then we'd write it down on a little note, stick it on the closet door, and repeat the message on a stickie on the mirror in the bathroom. They then had reinforced messages to calm them.

"Very often we found that writing a loving message and posting it on the door of their room or a closet gave them a lift as well."

Joanne: "My children would do that whenever they visited Poppy or Marnie. They'd leave little notes for them to find after they had left. It made them so happy."

Rita: "I very much like what that kindness does to the character of our children at the same time!"

### * Use of Family Albums

Joanne: "Do you remember telling me about your use of family albums with confused or distraught loved ones?"

Rita: "Yes, that's another technique which has worked well. When the people at the retirement home became frightened by their thoughts, I would bring out their family album. Family members would supply these to us upon our request. I would open to some picture that I guessed or knew was very special to the resident. Then I would attempt to engage the resident in conversation about it."

Joanne: "The pictures would trigger the stories that made them feel in touch again."

Rita: "That's right. Often their long-term memories were extremely clear and being able to call up memories was satisfying to them."

Joanne: "So to review the practical ways to alleviate the normal anxiety of our vulnerable loved ones, we need to keep in mind their essential humanity. Just as we get tense and upset in our much more fulfilling lives, so too will older people feel pressured in their changed patterns of life."

Rita: "We can help them and ourselves by using clarity cards, memory aids like the stickies, using their ability to read late into life, family albums, and any other creative ideas which can ease the difficulties of reduced capability.

"Most important of all will be our commitment to seeing our elderly relatives and friends not as annoying, demanding intrusions in our nice, neat lives but as valued people of diminished capacity."

Joanne: "... who can be helped by a creative approach and a compassionate spirit."

Rita: "Exactly."

## 4. *TONE, TOUCH AND TRANSITION*

Joanne: "When you first told me about using family albums to ease the fearful or angry patient in your nursing home, you showed by example another important method of easing anxiety. You actually repeated the conversation with which you would try to encourage them in this process.

"I was so struck by how beautifully you spoke: your tone of voice, the use of loving terms of endearment, and your choice of words were so moving."

Rita: "You call that nonverbal communication, don't you?"

Joanne: "Yes, in my consulting business and in dozens of college classes, I have taught that the use of thoughtful nonverbal communication can work wonders in a situation. I must say your use of nonverbal communication showed great mastery."

Rita: "Thank you. It's nice to get a compliment from a professional."

Joanne: "Well deserved and for such a good cause."

## * Nonverbal Communication works

Rita: "There's no question that it's important to allow the sound of your voice (paralanguage) and your use of certain tones ('Everything's fine.') to carry the message that 'all is well' and 'remember how happy your life has been.' At the same time, your touches (tactile communication) are saying: 'don't be afraid' through hugs and gestures."

Joanne: "Experts stress that nonverbal communication is perceived as more credible than verbal messages. For example, if a person compliments another with flowery and flattering words, yet shows no smile or approval on the face, usually that compliment will not be believed. On the other hand, an approving facial expression when giving critical feedback can take the negative sting out of it when done right."

Rita: "I believe that."

Joanne "Never is this more true than when working with the elderly. You have told me that their ability to translate nonverbal communication persists long after they cannot decipher human speech. In fact, I have seen the truth of this in my own family."

Rita: "As I have in mine."

Joanne: "Facial expressions are particularly communicative."

Rita: "Yes, it's true. The unfortunate thing is that sometimes it's so difficult to maintain our composure while performing the hard work of nursing care that our faces become set with concentration and our loved ones see that as disapproving of them. Occasionally one will see this in childcare as well; the overworked parent trying too hard to be perfect and communicating unintended messages to the child by facial expression."

Joanne: "I've been guilty of that, too. But to get back to our conversation, are there any other examples of nonverbals you'd like to tell us about?"

### *Environment counts*

Rita: "It goes beyond tone, body language, touch, even facial expressions. The *environment* surrounding the older person also gives them messages: for example, the old chair that once held a young mother and her new baby carries those memories with it when that mother is eighty and furnishing an assisted-living apartment. That chair should go with her into that apartment.

"A piece of jewelry given by a beloved friend — special music selections — a little painting of a familiar scene — notes and cards from family and friends: all these things should have a place in the home environment of the elderly person."

Joanne: "Just think how influenced we are, you and I, when there are three days of rain in a row. That gloomy environment affects our outlook on life and perhaps even our relationships with others. So a stark, stripped down room in which an elderly person resides can cause a lowering of spirits to follow."

Rita: "An effort needs to be made to decorate the living space of older people with their memories and needs and emotions in mind. Color, sound, access, safety, privacy: all these issues should be considered to communicate the supportive climate we wish for our loved ones. I guess you could call this nonverbal communication of the spatial kind."

## *Recommendations for Positive Nonverbal Communication with Elderly Loved Ones*

### Paralanguage:

(Tone of voice, pace of speech, volume, positive word choice)

Greetings are particularly important; make them warm and friendly, using an appropriate name for the older person. Determine whether the lady or man wants to be called by first name or title and/or last name, i.e., Ann or Mrs. Mary or Dr. Thompson or Grandpa.

Be aware of the sounds your voice makes. Does your tone carry a positive connotation? Does it sound happy, respectful, approving? Are you speaking too rapidly to be followed? Be sure to speak loudly enough and slowly enough for a person with some hearing loss to be able to understand you. In some cases, the older person will no longer bother to say: "I can't hear you." So the message delivered gets lost and becomes the cause of misunderstanding.

Try to ask for cooperation on a task rather than telling them to do it; for example, "Would you take along these towels for your bath? Thanks." Write your messages when there's a chance they won't be remembered or completely understood. Even delusional people can still read but can rarely remember instructions for more than a few minutes. However, this way they can re-read and reinforce the message. Then too, written messages of approval can give pleasure to your loved one: "You look handsome today."

Compliments are a wonderful treat for anyone but especially for someone who hears so few. Older people may protest and disagree when compliments are offered, but they warm their hands over the kind words after they are spoken. And of course, there is nothing better than being told that someone loves them. That's the highest form of positive word choice.

## **Body Language:**
(Positioning, facial expressions, stance, gestures, eye contact)

Since many older people have hearing losses, try to position yourself on the side with the better hearing or the ear with a hearing aid. Keep yourself turned to them so they can see your lips form the words and connect with your facial expressions. Cataracts or Macular Degeneration symptoms in the early stages do limit vision; so keeping close enough to be seen while talking helps to overcome the stress somewhat.

Of course, the most compelling means of communicating by body language is through facial expressions. An infant can recognize faces very early in life; an elderly person carries years of recognition skills to each communication. Use this ability of theirs by smiling, looking interested, acting pleased, or any other approving behaviors to enhance your relationship and demonstrate the value of the other person.

Even stance and gestures can indicate acceptance and affection. Holding hands while speaking or touching a cheek, when appropriate, can make an older person feel liked and worthwhile. For many elderly, days can go by without the touch of a human hand or the sense of someone standing near. Yet we are community-oriented creatures who really need this contact.

Probably the strongest point of contact is through the eyes. When someone is aged and still rational, he or she is quite aware of the personal loss of what is commonly accepted as beauty in the world. As a result, the old are extremely conscious of their appearance and acknowledge that many people avert their eyes when in their presence.

Instead, concerned caregivers should direct their eye contact very deliberately to the faces of their care recipients to reinforce their acceptance and approval of these people. This eye contact coupled with good facial expressions can work wonders for the self esteem and self confidence of the older persons under their care.

Steady eye contact can help to quiet anxiety and depression as well. In fact, when one looks deeply into the face of a loved one, one can not help but be moved and warmed by the deeper beauty written there by the presence of character and sacrifices of life.

## **Tactile Communication:**
(Touch, affectionate movement, sensory stimulation)

Most important point — if the older care recipient was a "touchy-feely" communicator throughout his or her life, then this tactile form of communication should be continued. If the person never seemed comfortable with displays of affection or demonstrativeness, they are unlikely to welcome it at this point in their lives. So a handshake rather than a hug for the latter person and kisses and pats for the former should fit the needs of both.

Touch is perhaps second only to eye contact as a strongly influential communication device. Experiments in the communication field demonstrate that since touch is the first of our responses to the presence of others while in infancy, it has strong psychological impact. Why not use it then to impart caring and calm and approval in our relations with older people?

**Some suggestions:** holding on to the waist while walking outside on a pleasant day; brushing his/her hair; giving a manicure; wrapping a soft blanket around chilly knees; offering a backrub; applying dry skin lotion; putting lipstick on a lady's lips; putting bubble bath into the bathtub; washing hair with a fragrant shampoo; placing a drop of perfume or after-shave lotion on the neck; dancing together to an old familiar song.

With the invalided or bedridden patient, choose bedding, pillows, covers, or blankets with great care to assure their softness and non-abrasive quality. Lifting the sheet, parachute fashion, and allowing air to envelope the resting person, can give a nice sensation when repeated for a few minutes.

It cools nicely and feels good as well — as do cool, wet cloths applied to the forehead or arms. Of course, air conditioning or fans make a world of difference. Many have mentioned the comfort of a sheepskin pad, too.

## **Spatial Communication**:
(Color, space, environment)

No matter what time of life one is experiencing, our surroundings always affect how we feel about our world and even ourselves. This is very true of the elderly person, especially when there's been a dislocation of his or her life. A new place. A new way of life. A different pattern of eating and sleeping and recreating. Attention should be paid to this aspect of an older person's world.

All of us have preferences when it comes to color. We ask little kids "What's your favorite color?" in an effort to show how special they are to us. Mightn't it be good idea to ask the same question of our older friends and family when we're decorating or painting their living quarters? Where possible, participation in choices for their walls and trim and fabric will give them a sense of freedom and importance. These choices communicate your respect for their opinions while allowing color selection which will give the greatest pleasure to your loved ones.

For those unable to make choices, of course, you will make the decisions for them to create aurroundings as comfortable and bright as possible, like including a favorite piece of furniture, pictures of family and friends, a handmade pillow, a place for notes and cards and seasonal events, and the use of colors that you remember they liked in their active lives.

Little things can also help ease their lives: the use of colored soaps so that when they are dropped, the soap can be seen against the white tub; installing a hand-held shower which allows the person to shower while seated on a water-proof stool in the shower stall; magnifying glasses (hand-held or electronic) for those whose sight is failing; books-on-tape to help pass the time for visually impaired people; shower caps to preserve hair styles while bathing.

The arrangement of furniture, presence of good lighting (sunshine and electric), absence of barriers

— all need to be considered as well in setting up the healthiest spatial environment. Just as a cold, dark room would clamp down on your spirit and emotions, so would it be for them. Your thoughtfulness in these matters makes space a way of telling your elderly residents that you care about them. It is a fine way of showing compassion.

In fact, let us consider separately just what it would be like to put ourselves in the place of our elderly for a few minutes to determine what our own basic needs would be were we uprooted from our familiar lives and moved into another's home. Since all of us hope to be old one day, this will be an exercise as much for ourselves as for our elderly loved ones.

## *Put yourself in their place*

What quality of life would be required to allow this person to be content and peaceful and perhaps even happy in a new environment? What does this older person need in the new home to achieve the satisfaction we all desire in our lifestyles? To answer we must be aware that these requirements will vary from person to person; however, there are some minimums that need to be considered.

Following is a list of some basic and beyond basic requirements that come to mind. Of course, there are more which you could identify.

## BASICS:
*a private place
*easy availability to food
*safe bathroom access, even at night
*warmth and quiet
*place for clothing
*local medical care
*daily contact with others
*hobby materials like a small garden or window box for a gardener or accommodation for stamp collecting or ceramic crafts or knitting or crochet
*a television set and radio and clock


## BASIC PLUS: when the person can no longer drive
*means of transportation — jitney bus, Senior van, car pooling, public bus as long as it is appropriate for this person's capabilities, taxis, friend's car
*rides to Bridge or Bingo or craft activities
*rides to church or temple or their activities
*rides to charity or volunteer work

*company on walks in the neighborhood

## *WELL BEYOND BASIC:*
*family gatherings to celebrate special events in the lives of elderly folks
*regular visits to old friends from different neighborhoods
*membership in exercise clubs
*weekly outings for shopping, hair care, flower or gift purchases, library visits, art classes, suitable movies
*trips to cultural events, concerts, elderhostel activities, art galleries, plays
*dining out from time to time with family or friends
*walking tours of historic neighborhoods

Joanne: "Well, that is a pretty comprehensive overview."

Rita: "What we want to do here is help spark thinking for caregivers."

Joanne: "For most readers, I suspect they'll read those lists and realize just what a good job they are doing for their loved ones; you know, saying 'Oh, I do that for Mom' or "I take Uncle Ted to Bingo every Thursday night." Nothing could give us more pleasure than lifting the spirits of these hard-working caregivers. These suggestions just emphasize that caregivers really need to be aware of the importance of nonverbal communication with their elderly."

Rita: "I remember your sharing with me your nonverbal experience with your mother, who understood your smiles and warm voice tones long after she had lost comprehension."

Joanne: "That meant the world to me, Rita. It kept a loving bond alive even when she didn't know my name or my relationship to her. Yet she expressed that she loved me at the end of her life and I believe she knew she was loved as well."

Rita: "And after her death, since you had managed to keep bonding through the difficult years, it seemed to help soften your grief."

### * Live in the absolute present

Joanne: "No question about that. It felt like I had been giving her up by inches but loving her every bit of the way. Afterward, I had no regrets.

There was also something important I came to know during those dark days that really helped me cope with her growing senility."

Rita: "You found something good in the midst of all that sadness?"

Joanne: "Yes, I really did. My mother had always been a world-class worrier. When there was little or no reason to be upset about an impending event, she could worry herself up one side and down the other. Throughout my life, I would scold her about that."

Rita: "Of course, that did no good whatsoever."

Joanne: "None at all. However, as she slid into increasing senility and non-comprehension, she also tended to become more calm. Her memory loss, once she no longer was aware of it, actually became a blessing. She had no fears, no negative projections, no unhappiness She was unable to worry about tomorrow's problems, nor could she regret anything in the past."

Rita: "In effect, she was forced to live in the absolute present! As long as she was surrounded by smiling people, warmth and good food, and given reassurance, she was at peace in the truest sense of that word."

Joanne: "Exactly. What is so ironic here is that living in the present is just what our world's greatest religions have been telling us to do."

Rita: "Yes, you and I really should try it sometime."

Joanne: "Well, when I finally stopped mourning *my loss* of Mom's active, funny, vital self and started concentrating on what was actually going on with her, I realized the mercy of the situation.

"In that mental state, with the exception of those moments of agitation or negative confusion, she was truly content, perhaps for the first time in her long life.

"For me, this was a new way of looking at things. It altered my thinking substantially and, in the process, gave me a great deal of comfort and acceptance of this life situation."

Rita: "Later on, I thought you found a wonderful way to help your father to change *his* way of looking at things."

## *\* A Life Transition*

Joanne: "You mean the letter Ed and I wrote to Dad?"

Rita: "Yes. I thought it really helped to ease his transition from his house to your home."

Joanne: "Well, my heart went out to him when in his late eighties it became apparent that Dad should no longer live alone. He simply couldn't keep things together any more, and we became very worried about him.

"Interestingly, when we spoke to him on the phone, he always sounded perfectly able to do everything. However, when we went and spent a weekend with him, then we knew otherwise."

Rita: "Yes, all their memory tracks are in place while speaking on the phone. They are better skilled in coping devices in that limited medium and can disguise a great deal."

Joanne: "It was a shock to see the difference between how he sounded and how he really was."

Rita: "My mother-in-law convinced all of us in her family that everything was great — over the phone. And just like your experience, it was a whole other story when we spent several days with her."

Joanne: "I remember that. You were so upset. In our case, once we saw the handwriting on the wall, we recognized that there had to be a change in his living arrangements; so, we wrote a letter to him proposing a new life for him."

"It began with a 'what if?' scenario and then described what his life with us could be like. We had done our homework and knew about all the services available for older people in our community.

"We'd worked out where his rooms would be; how he could meet new friends; what recreation was available for him; all of that. Then we used words to paint a picture of him in a calm, secure, and loving environment."

Rita: "How did you give it to him?"

Joanne: "Ed and I went to his house for the day and we made a formal presentation to him in his living room."

Rita: "Did it upset him?"

Joanne: "When he read it, he cried. Then he said: 'This is a beautiful letter.' We told him to read it over for the next week and that we would return to hear his answer.

"When we came back, the next Sunday, he said: 'Yes, I'll come. It's the only logical thing to do.' Since then he has made a terrific transition, and frankly, just in the nick of time."

Rita: "A very humane approach to a difficult life change."

Joanne: "Thank you. I'm including the letter even though we're aware that every circumstance would be different. It's just to help give readers some idea of what worked so well for us."

### * *"Imagine a Man Who..." Letter*

*October 22, xxxx*

*Dear Dad,*

*There's an invitation for you which I will tell you about at the end of this letter, but first I want to paint a picture which might help you to answer.*

*I see a man in my imagination and I would like you to imagine him too.*

*I see a man living his life pretty much as he is living it now, without the anxiety of debt, taxes, isolation, and occasional fear. His family loves him very much and wants what is best for him, especially freedom from pressing financial matters. This family wants to join him helpfully in the sometimes difficult later years of his life. He has been supportive of so many others, it is not surprising that his family wants to participate in supporting him now.*

*I see this man in a comfortable, private apartment in the lower half of his only daughter's home, a carpeted, warm living room, an adjacent activity room/kitchen for his projects, a separate bedroom, and a bathroom. His own furniture would be there, TV and all, arranged around a fireplace in the living room. The door between upstairs and his apartment would be opened or closed as the spirit moved him.*

*I see a man with absolutely no financial problems: no need to pay for house upkeep, rent, heating or lighting, or any other home expense. A man whose debts have been paid off and who can use the*

*Social Security check he collects for his own purposes only. This man can eat alone or with his family as he wishes. He can do his own shopping or raid his family's refrigerator. He can enjoy his daughter's cooking or his own — his choice.*

*I see a man who is with his immediate and extended family for all the major holidays, not 80 miles away on the other side of impossible traffic. This man would continue to visit with the friends of his later years on a frequent basis while his daughter visits her friends, too.*

*I see a man in a community with an active senior adults club, which offers a hot lunch every day as well as occasional outings in the community-owned Senior Bus. This bus picks up members in front of their homes daily and for free.*

*There is a church in this community, just eight minutes from home. There's an outreach program like the one you so enjoy where groceries are shared with less fortunate people every week. They're looking for volunteers. There's a hospital nearby which uses older people as volunteers as well.*

*This is the picture as I believe it could be lived, — a safer, friendlier, more protected family environment for this man, whom I have always loved. If this man would consent to join his family in mid-December, he could spend Christmas with them in his pretty new apartment or wait until after Christmas if that would suit him better.*

*You are that man and this could be your new life.*

*I recognize the sacrifice of such a difficult life change, but I also know that your sound mind and good health make this change possible and peaceful at this time, — whereas we none of us know what the future might bring. Moving an older person because of a health crisis makes for a far more heartbreaking and fearful life event. It would be so much better to see this reunion as a happy challenge with a tear in the eye and a smile on the face.*

*So, my recommendation is this: Come and live with us. Come and be close family with us at a time in our joint lives when we know how precious every day must be. Aren't you a little afraid of the future, too?*

*Wouldn't it be nice to watch an occasional ballgame with Ed, down in your apartment? Wouldn't it be fun to help us decorate our Christmas tree next year up in the living room? (You can hang the tinsel; no one has ever done it better.) Wouldn't it be pleasant to meet some new friends up here in our town while keeping in touch with your old friends? And wouldn't it be nice to be more deeply involved in the lives of your family's children at closer range?*

*I will ask you now to think long and hard about this recommendation, and next Sunday, we will ask you for your decision. We'll come to you then and hear what you've decided.*

*Know that we love you, we want you, and your decision is important to all of us.*

*All our Love,*

*Joanne, Ed and the Family*

# 5. *FORGIVE OUR TRESPASSES*

## * Nobody's Perfect

Joanne: "You know, Rita, we might be guilty of creating a false impression."

Rita: "Like what?"

Joanne: "Since our conversation is almost 100% hindsight, we could be giving the false idea that we knew what we were doing all the time we were doing it."

Rita: "If only that could have been the case!"

Joanne: "Exactly. So much of what I did was heartbreaking trial and error. I don't know what I would have done without your advice during those tough years with first my mother's care and then my father's."

Rita: "It was only through trial and error that I learned enough to be able to advise you, and the bad part about trial and error are all the errors you commit while undergoing the trial part. When it's live human beings in the mix, it's a complicated and emotional business. Many times we said to each other: 'Do the best you can' and that was all we had."

Joanne: "On some really bad days, that became a mantra. Okay, we made mistakes. Let's just remember: Love is learning to say you're sorry. And I said a lot of those, not only to my parents but much more to my four kids in their growing-up years and beyond.

Rita: "Oh, don't start on the kids too! I won't sleep tonight!"

Joanne: "Listen to you — I used to envy the calm and steady way you worked with your five kids. I took so much good example from you."

Rita: "You didn't know what was going on inside me to give that impression."

Joanne: "You'll never convince me otherwise. But to get back to my point: caregivers must realize that mistakes will be made and not only by us, but by our elderly care recipients. This is a very inexact process and allowances must be made for the humanity of our collaboration. Forgiveness has got to be part of the deal or we're finished."

Rita: "Such a good point, Joanne. And the forgiveness goes both ways:

forgive ourselves for our errors in judgment or emotion, and forgive our parents for their mistakes in raising us as well."

### *Old wrongs, old hurts*

Joanne: "In some cases, those mistakes have been devastating: the father who ran out on the family years before, the mother who drank, Uncle Willie who stole from a relative. Heavy duty mistakes."

Rita: "Mistakes which might require extraordinary character if one is to be a caregiver to that person. It's tough enough performing the caregiving, but when there are other deep-rooted issues as well, then decisions need to be made.

"Can the caregiver forgive the elderly person? Will smoldering resentment intrude day by day? Can the vulnerability and fragility of the old person overcome the natural resistance of a wronged daughter or son?"

Joanne: "While there is no way we can advise in these horribly difficult circumstances, we do know that an aged lady or man must be overseen. If someone's hatred of that person, no matter how justified, is going to get in the way of healthy day-to-day care, some other person or agency must be called into the picture. It is inhumane treatment of the elderly if the angry feelings can't be left outside the situation."

Rita: "It is of course true that some incredible people have risen above very natural reactions to harsh or even brutal treatment in their early lives and still find it in their hearts to extend mercy to elderly relatives in their care."

Rita: "God bless those heroes. Just the same, retribution cannot be a factor in caring for the elderly. The old person has the law, social judgment, and even the Ten Commandments on his or her side; anything with the appearance of neglect or maltreatment becomes abuse if Social Services gets involved. As a result, the caregiver has to be able to act toward the old person in a consistently positive manner if they take on that awesome responsibility."

## *What not to do*

Joanne: "When I want to conjure up a point of reference in my mind for what not to do with an elderly relative or friend, I recall an experience I had when my husband, Ed, and I were members of the Parish Mission Team in New York City. We would give missions for four days a week in local parishes, sharing our experiences with members of the community."

Rita: "I remember that very well."

Joanne: "That's right — we came to *your* church that spring. And do you recall how we went to the homes of some of the infirm elderly parishioners to visit and pray with them?"

Rita: "Yes, I got to go with you on a couple of visits!"

Joanne: "Well, several months later, Ed and I went to a home in another parish where we saw the opposite of everything you and I saw in your parish visits — and everything we are recommending in these conversations.

"In this home there was a woman in her mid-seventies who lived on the lower level of a high ranch.  She had her own kitchen, living room, bath and bedroom on her level, and her son and his family were on the second level with a self-contained private apartment.  I suspect the house was owned by the woman we were visiting; she had perhaps invited her son to move in and care for her in return for his housing.

She had the worst case of arthritis I had ever seen, causing her constant pain and confining her to a wheelchair for most of the time.  But I think the greater pain was in her soul.

"All the doors between her apartment and theirs were shut tight.  Food was delivered twice a day from upstairs with no interaction.  Her grandchildren were kept away, and her isolation was complete.

"As we chatted and prayed with her, she sobbed non-stop.  She spoke of her pain and sadness and loneliness.  We were devastated.  As outsiders, we certainly couldn't directly affect the situation by talking with the woman's son, but our parish guide, a Catholic sister, did promise that she would see what could be done to ease this woman's isolated situation."

Rita:  "It breaks your heart to see that kind of alienation.  Sometimes in my hospice work, I stumble into that kind of thing. It is as if people are meeting the letter of the law but not its spirit. We humans need community and we need a purpose. Otherwise it's like living in solitary confinement."

Joanne: "Now it's important to remember that we did not know the whole story here. It is very possible that there might have been baggage from the past influencing the young couple to act as they did, or some early issues about which we knew nothing."

Rita: "Yes, that does happen. People endure child abuse or alcoholic episodes or other crises and they become bitter. It 's very hard to blame the grown children for being unwilling to care for a parent who failed them in their youth."

Joanne: "Exactly. Maybe that had happened in this case, maybe not. The fact remains that the older person needs help now, in this time, and the child needs to deal with the overwhelming need of the care recipient no matter what."

Rita: "Very hard to do. The Good Lord has the answer but it's not an answer easily performed."

Joanne: "Forgive, forgive, forgive into infinite numbers?"

Rita: "That's the idea."

Joanne: "What a tough problem for those coming from really bad backgrounds. I would propose a few sessions with a psychologist or a therapist as a good start in those cases. Yet I think it's always hard, even for those of us with pretty good familial backgrounds."

Rita: "That's what I've seen through the years in the nursing home — many normal family groups with lots of dysfunction in the past and present.

So just about all of us have to find ways to forgive our parents for being imperfect. Ed Hughes wrote about that for us in this poem."

How much care is needed
        for a senior who is ailing?
How much understanding
        heals an elder who is failing?

How many spurs of memory
        cause our gratitude to start?
How many hugs and kisses
        thank an old and trembling heart?

## FORGIVE OUR TRESPASSES

How much compassion flows
        for loss of every vital sense?
How much love and patience
        can we give aging residents?

*As much as we can manage*,
        the answer's from on high;
As we love one another,
        that's as much as we should try.

Rita: "I think you could add another line:

'How much to forgive a parent?
        As much as they might need it.'

Joanne: "And *our* kids will have to forgive us for *our* human failings! Maybe each of us should spend some time figuring out how all of us can do this repetitive forgiving. I say repetitive because life teaches us that that is the nature of forgiving— once is never enough."

# 6.  *MAKE SOMEONE HAPPY*

## * *Eighty-year-old hands*

A personal note from Joanne on the theme of this chapter:

"When I visited my mother's home one day late in her life, we were talking in her kitchen. She was all dressed up for the visit and she accepted my compliments on how nice she looked. Then she started shaking her head in exasperation as she looked down at her hands. 'I just don't know what to do about my hands, Joanne; they look so old,' she said.

"I glanced at her soft and wrinkled hands as she stated: 'They look like 80-year-old hands!' Then she stopped, looked up at me, and said:
'Oh, that's right — I *am* eighty!'

"We both laughed so hard we were bent double.

"When I remember my deceased mother, it is that wonderful laugh we had together that invariably puts a smile back on my face . She was so much fun and so responsive to others. That hilarious moment brings her back to me as she was in life.

"We must keep the laughter in our lives — as long as those lives might last. For the loved one, it is humanizing and endearing; for those of us who give the care, it's a lifesaver.

"With the help of some friends in the business of caring for the elderly, Rita and I have compiled some recommendations which might lighten the load by which eldercare sometimes burdens us. Hope they help."

### * *Family thoughtfulness*

Anytime several family members can be involved in caring for their older relatives or family friends, it is good for them and miraculous for the older person.

——-**Give a family gift** of a VCR to care recipients, then encourage the sending of copies of family activity videos to them. It keeps them in the loop of birthdays, holidays, etc. and allows them to respond by phone or note to the kindness, keeping communication open on both sides.

————**-Interview the older person** by video or audio as to their memories of their childhood or early years and their perceptions of your own early years. It is wonderful to see this done by a teenager or older child, again for both sakes.

————**-Have family members e-mail** their positive remembrances of grandparents or older relatives to a central location, print them out, assemble in a scrapbook and give them to the lucky person. Use larger font if eyesight is poor. Have this scrapbook available at the next family gathering so that everyone can see the kind words and sweet memories of the loved one.

————**-Ask an elderly person** who is capable to put together an album of pictures for a young family. Buy a fresh scrapbook or album, supply the pictures (previously numbered), and some decorative materials (stickers, ribbons, or used greeting cards to cut flowers or words from to serve as borders or pretty effects.) This will earn praise for the "artist" and a needed boost for the busy young parent.

————**-Make a plan** to have everyone in the family call the loved one on a special day, breaking the day into timeframes that make the calls more convenient for callers. For example, the family in California will love to call late in the day if they're calling the East Coast, but won't welcome a wake-up call at four, their time.

————-**Get family members together** for a brainstorming session on "Making the Bathroom Safer and More Comfortable for _____ (Granny, Uncle Ned, Grandpa, or other)." Talk about and then implement changes like removing all loose rugs, installing hand rails, putting in a night light, getting a waterproof stool with rubber cups on the legs for seating during a shower, and all the other good ideas the group can imagine. It not only helps the care receiver but gives relatives a chance to share with you and the older person. Always a good thing.

————-**At major events, nominate a seasonal "chair"** to make a special day for the older person, i.e., younger sister Susie will take Grandma to a Memorial Service for Uncle John every October or son-in-law Hank will buy tickets to a Yankee Game for Dad once a year in baseball season. This cuts through the "I'm too busy" syndrome since everyone is pitching in to do one thing a year, especially if it's an occasion in which they have some self interest.

We're sure if you and your family members get together once in a while and raise this issue of creative kindness for an elderly person who needs this love from you so much, there will be dozens of ideas far better then these. Give it a try. With a little luck , it may become addictive.

### * A little gardening

So often, the infirmity of old age closes off some of the activities that made life worth living to many people. If a person has been a lifelong gardener, it is so sad to see this skilled experience unused. But in so many cases, arthritic fingers, swollen knees, hurting backs can't manage the pain active gardening can cause and the participation ceases.

We'd like to suggest some alternative forms of gardening which can be pursued without the difficulties of normal landscape or vegetable gardening around the house. Let them trigger your own creativity.

————-**Hanging baskets can be placed** within arm's length of even the most disabled older person with the opportunity to deadhead the flowers and mist them each day. Tiny watering devices can be placed conveniently to allow this gentle care. The pleasure received can be so satisfying — both to the gardener and to you for thinking of it.

———-**Window boxes too can offer** a suitable framework for not-so-nimble fingers. Yet to be able to choose the annual flowers that will dress the box, plant them, fertilize from time to time, pick off the dead blooms, and water every few days — well, that's just plain fun! Of course, your help and transportation might be needed, although I doubt your advice will.

———-**Sometimes the older gardener simply needs some help** with the weeding and manual work. The gift of a young neighbor's effort for four hours, pre-paid, might be much more appreciated than a birthday blouse.

———-**The older active person might volunteer** to help with some municipal gardens (gardens under the welcoming signs for a town, sidewalk cut-out gardens, barrels of flowers planted by civic organizations, etc.) They are not so demanding as a whole backyard and so pleasing to the community.

————-**Encourage the growing of  wonderful indoor plants** like orchids or cyclamens for a dramatic floral change of pace.  There are loads of recommendations for their care, even Orchid Societies ready to advise.

————-If all else fails, **think about a weekly gift of fresh flowers** for the older person to arrange, supplying materials to make this possible, or a windowsill herb garden for the kitchen.    It provides a ready source of conversational material which is fresh and reality based, rather than a long recitation of complaints or illnesses.   Good for them, good for you.

## *\* Devices that can help*

It can be useful to pore over the dozens of catalogs that many of us receive weekly to see if there might be some offerings that can put a smile on the face of our care receivers or provide safety aid.   Rita and I managed to find the following; we're sure you can do even better.

————-Jigsaw puzzles with large enough pieces for swollen fingers to handle.

———-Big playing cards, easy to hold and easy to read.

———-Earphones so that volume can be loud yet silent to others.

———-Support furniture for incapacitated elderly like

~gerry chairs (with trays that come over in front and prevent the person from getting up until safety is assured),

~beds that raise up both top and bottom,

~chairs that lift the person to a standing position,

~the "Merry Walker" which provides lightweight surrounding support for walking and a flat seat in back for a quick sit-down if required,

~canes and walkers when stability becomes tenuous,

~next-to-the-bed chairs with removable pots to help with nighttime bathroom calls.

Many of these devices can be purchased in medical supply stores or through catalogs for the sick or elderly.

————-Bright lights with flexible necks for good positioning while reading.

————-Walker-like grocery carts for those who walk to their shopping sites.

————-Wire frames that can support books or magazines on a desk for reading without holding the weight of the volume in the hands.

————Velcro closure strips for shoes, clothing, hats, for convenience.

————-**Make up a big Calendar** on oaktag cardboard and place it in your loved one's room. Every day cross off the day just lived and write in any special day coming up in clear lettering. Make it seasonal and holiday-oriented.

Use pictures of snow and mountains and flowers and fruits and babies and multi-environmental references to keep him or her in touch with the world.

————-**Show videos from the past on a VCR** : Abbot and Costello, *I Love Lucy*, The Milton Berle Show, Busby Berkeley musicals, movies from the thirties and forties, etc., Jerry Lewis movies, cartoons, Disney offerings.

———-**Seek out Books on Tape** for the sight impaired person.    Many communities have volunteers who read weekly over the radio for those who have trouble seeing fine print.    The libraries have many selections of these helpful books.

———-**Elderhostels are college-sponsored educational packages** for older people who want to continue educating themselves.    They are geared to safety, intellectual stimulation, and appropriate accommodations.    Contact a local college for names of sponsoring institutions and dates.

———-**Elderly residents enjoy participation** in their local   school plays, concerts, and sports events.    Watch the newspapers for announcements of these inexpensive or free offerings.

———-**Golden Agers and Senior Olympians keep young** and love company. Posters, handouts, and press releases keep communities informed of their activities.    All are welcome.

———-For more good ideas in the laughter department, write to *The Humor Project,* **480 Broadway, Ste. 210, Saratoga Springs, New York 12866** for materials that are designed to help caregivers find humor in what they do. Phone: 518-587-8770 or www.HumorProject.com.

## 7. *WHERE TO LOOK FOR HELP*

### * *Some research tools*

When home care is entered into, there are agencies and support groups to aid in this important and often courageous undertaking. Become a student of this research, reading all you can find and searching through newspapers and magazines and on the search engines of the Internet to get as much data as you can to help you in this invaluable work.

From *Parade Magazine*, July 16, 2000 issue, from the article titled "How Can We Help?" by Bernard Gavzer, page 4. Reprinted with permission from *Parade*, copyright c 2000.

———-Require a health-care aide?
Free brochure *How to Choose a Home Care Provider*, write to the National Association for Home Care Dept. P, 228 Seventh Avenue, S.E., Washington, D.C. 20003

————-Need an afternoon off?

Check out local hospitals, friends, your church, adult care programs, family members, county offices for the aging for volunteers to give you an occasional break. See your local Phone Book for the **Office for the Aging**.

————-Facing a catastrophe?

*Parade Magazine* reports on the ***Family Medical Leave Act of 1993***. This act gives employees the chance to take up to 12 weeks of unpaid leave a year to care for an elderly relative. Talk to your employer. In an emergency, siblings might be able to share caregiving by staggering these unpaid weeks of leave whereby no one is out of work for very long periods, but this special care is given a week at a time by several loved ones.

————-Need a professional caregiver?

Look in your local phone book for **Visiting Nurse Agencies**, which offer non-profit, home-based care for your elderly relatives or friends.

To get a good overview, write ***Visiting Nurse Associations of America* 11 Beacon Street, Dept. P, Suite 910, Boston, MA 02108**

## *\* If Home Care becomes impossible*

When health crises strike our elderly, some alternatives are available.

————-**Local Hospitals** can offer the medical care your care receiver might need. However, we strongly recommend your active involvement as an Advocate for your loved one in this environment. Overworked and understaffed health care providers can slide an old person to the bottom of their priority list. Be there very often to make sure your family members or friends don't lose out on the care they deserve. Act in a friendly and helpful manner but don't be afraid to ask for and even insist on what is necessary.

————-A **Nursing Home** may be needed <u>short-term</u> for recovery after a broken hip or a wound that won't heal or <u>long-term</u> after a major stroke and/or devastating surgery. These skilled nursing care facilities are for those with the most demanding needs. The hospital which has supervised your loved one's medical care will be a great resource for you in explaining the requirements for entry of your loved one into a nursing home.

———-If your care receiver doesn't require this skilled nursing care, but has come to the place where more constant oversight is necessary, your best bet might be from **Assisted Living** for the older person. This care usually affords an apartment-like setting with no stairs and maximum safety plus companionship to a greater or lesser degree.

———-Sometimes older people prefer a smaller, more intimate environment in a group with several other elderly titled **Adult Foster Care.** This costs less than the other two options and may be incorporated into the above situations. Of course, many other residential opportunities exist and should be investigated until an appropriate match is made.

———-For an overview of even **more alternatives,** write to Family Caregiver Alliance

690 Market Street, Dept. P., Suite 600
San Francisco, CA 94104
or visit their Website:
www/caregiver.org/factsheets/out_of_home
_care.htmi.

————-Still confused or uncertain about what to do when homecare cannot be given? Maybe a professional **Geriatric Caregiver** is what you need. Of course, there would be a fee for these services but it might fit your situation perfectly. There is a Website for the following:

> National Association of Geriatric Care Managers
> www.caremanager.org.

# 8. *EMPATHY IS EVERYTHING*

Please remember the earliest recommendation of this little book:
*Be empathic with your elderly.*

Put yourself in their place to aid in *your* understanding. There cannot be compassion without recognizing the human link between those who were born before us and ourselves.

The following poem appeared in the "Personal Look" section of ADVANCE for Nurse Practitioners, June 1993, Vol. 1, No. 3, page 22. It was contained in an article written by Steven D. Johnson, who teaches in the Primary Care Associate Program of Stanford University/Foothill Community College in Stanford, California.

With his permission, I quote: "...[this poem] was found in an elderly woman's locker after she died in a geriatric hospital. Each year I share the poem in my introductory lecture on Geriatric Care....The poem serves to remind me of my limited perception and helps me to respect the person for whom I perform my task. It keeps me honest and humble in the face of those who trust me with their care."

# A CRABBIT OLD WOMAN

What do you see, Nurse, what do you see?
What are you thinking when you're looking at me?
   A crabbit old woman, not very wise,
     Uncertain of habit, with faraway eyes,

Who dribbles her food and makes no reply
When you say in a loud voice, "I do wish you'd try."
   Who seems not to notice the things that you do,
     And forever is losing a stocking or shoe.

Who unresisting or not, lets you do as you will
With bathing, and feedings, the long days to fill.
   Is that what you're thinking?  Is that what you see?
     Then open your eyes, Nurse — you're not looking at me.

I'll tell you who I am as I sit here so still,
As I rise at your bidding — as I eat at your will.
   I'm a small child of ten with a father and mother,
     Brothers and sisters who love one another.

A young girl of sixteen with wings on her feet
Dreaming that soon now, a lover she'll meet.
   A bride soon at twenty — my heart gives a leap,
     Remembering the vows that I promised to keep.

At twenty-five now I have young of my own,
Who need me to build a secure, happy home.
   A woman of thirty, my young now grow fast,
     Bound to each other with ties that should last.

At forty, my young sons have grown up and are gone,
But my man's beside me to see I don't mourn.
   At fifty, once more babies play round my knee.
    Again, we know children, my loved one and me.

Dark days are upon me — my husband is dead.
I looked at the future, I shudder with dread,
   For my young are all rearing young of their own,
    And I think of the years and the love that I've known.

I'm an old woman now, and Nature is cruel —
"T'is her jest" to make old age look like a fool.
   The body is crumpled, grace and vigor depart —
    There is now a stone where I once had a heart.

But inside the carcass a young girl still dwells,
And now and again my battered heart swells.
   I remember the joys — I remember the pain,
    And I'm loving and living Life over again.

I think of the years — all too few —gone too fast,
And accept the stark fact that nothing can last.
   So open your eyes, Nurse, — open and see
    Not a Crabbit Old Woman — look closer — see me.

## * *A summary*

Rita: " I hope this helps those who are working so hard and lovingly with their elderly family or friends.

Joanne: "If it helps them even a little bit in the wonderful way you helped me with my mother and then my father, it will all have been worth the effort."

Rita: "I loved sharing that time with you and indirectly, with your parents."

**Joanne: "Wouldn't it be wonderful if people reading this book would let us know what has worked for them? "**

**Rita: "Let's invite them to write or e-mail us with their reactions to this book and to their own circumstances. In time, we might be able to publish their suggestions too, to help still more of the caregiving population. We'll put our address and e-mail on the last page."**

Joanne: "Well, some of these relationships with elderly people can be the most difficult in our lives. Often, it really requires help from outside the family just as you gave me, and it's amazing what a difference it can make. After all, most grown-ups are really rather good at what we do. We've lived a long time and usually have our acts together. And then along comes Grandma with a set of needs and requirements absolutely outside the area of expertise that most of us have developed — and we're beginners again."

Rita: "That's when friends can help."

Joanne: "Yeah, when they're knowledgeable friends like you, but oftentimes our family and friends don't know any more than we do."

Rita: "It's true; they don't always know enough to help that person to hang on to independence and humor with the necessary respect and affection."

Joanne: "And who of us can live without those qualities?"

Rita: "It becomes existing, not living, when that loving concern is not there."

Joanne: "Let's hope this book energizes some of the compassionate and giving caregivers out there and gives them credit and hope.

Rita: "I wish them well as I do their loved ones. They are doing such a significant and extremely difficult work. There's no doubt that it's occasionally hard to focus on the elderly person's need for love and affection. Their coping skills become so flawed that they aren't always loveable in their manner. Stick it out; it's worth it. Anne Landers has a column that encourages that idea so well, and we have her permission to use it as our last offering to caregivers."

## "The Time is Now"

If you are going to love me,
Love me now, while I can know
The sweet and tender feelings
Which from true affection flow.

Love me now while I am living,
Do not wait until I'm gone
And then have it struck in marble,
Tender words on ice-cold stone.

Do not wait until I sleep,
Tell me now your tender thoughts.
Don't let Death come between us
And sweet Love come to naught.

While we're living heart to heart,
Share with me a little bit.
If you love me, let me hear you;
So that I can treasure it.

With permission of Ann Landers, P.O. Box 11562,
Chicago, Ill.  606611-0562

# 9. *A PAGE OF THANKS*

To our husbands Edward: Miller and Hughes, who encouraged us not only in the writing of this small book, but by living lives of active compassion toward all our elderly loved ones.

To our parents, who gave such good example of caring for their elderly loved ones during the course of their lives: Dr. and Mrs. Alfred Imperato and Mr. and Mrs. Thomas Reilly. It is the late Mr. Reilly, Joanne Hughes' father, who is holding his great grand-daughter Emily Kern in the cover picture.

To Ann Landers, who let us use the poem, *The Time is Now.*

To Steven D. Johnson, who is an empathic teacher of caregivers, and who allowed us to use the poem that he shares with his nursing classes, *A Crabbit Old Woman.*

To *Parade Magazine*, which generously shared its information treasures on the resources for the elderly, and the author Bernard Gavzer, whose article "How Can We Help?" offers great insight into caring for the elderly person.

To the Humor Project, which wants to put a smile on the face of the world.

To Elizabeth, Thomas, Edward, John, and David Miller and their families and Elizabeth, Jennifer, Ted, and Allison Hughes and their families, who will be expected to memorize this book prior to taking on the care of the authors.

## 10.  *WILL YOU SHARE WITH US?*

If you'd like to communicate with us about your experiences with the elderly or offer your suggestions for working well with older people, write us or e-mail us at:  efxh@webtv.net

> or write us at:
> Mrs. Joanne Hughes
> c/o BCW Inc.
> P.O. Box  283
> Cornwall, New York 12815—0283

If you would like us to include your recommendation in this or future books, please attach a dated and signed statement releasing us from responsibility for liability or payment. Thanks so much.